I dedicate this book to David, Steven, Alan and my father Ken. Also in loving memory of my mother, Jeanne.

Published by
Venture Press, 16 Kent Street, Birmingham B5 6RD.

British Library Cataloguing-in-Publication Data.
A catalogue record for this book is available from the British Library.

ISBN 1 86178 066 4 (paperback).

Design, typesetting and printing by
Hobbs the Printers Limited, Brunel Road, Totton, Hampshire SO40 3WX.

Direct Payments:
practitioner's guide Series

Janet Leece

VENTURE PRESS

Contents

Acknowledgements

My grateful thanks to all those who have helped me to write this book: Jackie Averill, Anne and Mike Coyne, David Leece, Maureen Newman, Ken Sewell, Darren Statham, Peter Steel and last, but by no means least, Rob Wilson from the Rowan Organisation.

Also many thanks to the National Centre for Independent Living for their unfailingly prompt and helpful responses to my interminable requests for information.

Introduction

Direct payments are probably the most radical and exciting change to the delivery of social care since the implementation of the NHS and Community Care Act in 1993. They have tremendous potential to meet the needs of service users in creative and more effective ways than traditional service delivery. They enable individuals to achieve power, choice and control over the way their social care is delivered. Direct payments have also been shown to be a cheaper way of meeting people's social care needs.

Yet there are still relatively few people using direct payments, especially individuals who have a learning disability or mental ill health. Research points to practitioners' lack of enthusiasm about direct payments for the low take-up nationally. Fear of the unknown, insufficient information or training, worry about things going wrong, a reluctance to deal directly with money, concern that vulnerable people will be exploited, and a resistance to the idea that people want to and can successfully make their own care arrangements. All these may be contributing to practitioners' anxiety and preventing them offering direct payments.

This book aims to remove the fear and uncertainty surrounding direct payments by providing practitioners with the practical information, knowledge and skills to feel confident about offering direct payments and enabling service users to access them successfully. It also considers issues important for direct payment schemes, such as enabling service users with a cognitive or learning disability to demonstrate consent to a direct payment; the ability to manage a direct payment; how to support direct payment users; employing family members; and the difficulties in recruiting personal assistants. Situations are brought to life by the use of anonymous case studies.

Chapter one explains direct payments and discusses their background. It details the relevant legislation and provides an explanation of eligibility for direct payments. There is a discussion about the advantages and disadvantages, together with clarification on how a direct payment can be calculated.

Chapter two is concerned with the assessment process and the importance for practitioners of completing a truly needs-led assessment, which can then be translated into a cash amount. There is a detailed discussion about assessing disabled children and young people, carers, parents, young carers, and service users with care needs that fluctuate.

The problems of defining care that is 'substantial and regular', whether people can demonstrate consent and whether they will be able to manage a direct payment are considered.

Chapter three, entitled 'Supporting people to use direct payments' covers all the practical areas that it may be necessary for practitioners to know about when arranging a direct payment. Using supporting agencies, creating a job description, writing a contract of employment, recruiting a suitable personal assistant, interviewing, managing PAYE and National Insurance contributions, health and safety legislation, insurance and pensions.

In Chapter four, strategies for making direct payments work are considered. The change in culture required for direct payments where there is a relinquishing of local authority power and an acceptance of service users' rights to take risks in the pursuit of greater independence and control. Contingency planning to stop molehills turning into mountains, and how best to involve people from minority ethnic communities, people with learning disabilities, people with mental ill health and so on to enable them to gain access to direct payment schemes. Using funding from the Independent Living Funds and Health Authorities together with direct payments to increase the amount of money available to pay for social care are also considered.

Chapter five draws the threads of the book together and highlights the pivotal role practitioners play in the direct payments process. Direct payments have such enormous possibilities for disabled adults, children, carers and parents, so it is crucial that, as practitioners, we get it right.

'I have been released from my prison by my direct payment. I am back in charge. I am happy and I am free'

1 What are direct payments?

Direct payments are all about enabling service users and carers to have greater power, choice and independence in their lives. They are intended to empower individuals to have greater control and freedom to participate fully in society.

A direct payment is a payment made by a local authority to an eligible individual. The local authority makes the payment instead of arranging or providing services to meet the assessed needs of the person. Individuals then use the payment themselves to purchase services to meet their assessed needs. This may involve buying care from an agency, buying respite care or day services, becoming an employer and recruiting a personal assistant and so on. Most people choose to spend their direct payment on employing their own personal assistant, as this option gives them the most control, independence and flexibility.

A direct payment cannot be used to purchase permanent residential care, nor can it be used to buy services provided directly by a local authority. People can, however receive both a direct payment and services provided or purchased by the local authority, as part of their care package. For example, an individual could receive a direct payment to purchase their personal care and still receive direct service provision in the form of a day service place.

Background

Direct payments are not a new idea. Schemes operate throughout Europe in a variety of forms, all with a system of direct funding, either in cash or vouchers, which people then use to buy their own care. The concept originated in Canada in the 1970s, where a group of parents were determined that residential care was not the answer for their disabled children. They battled for the right to receive cash payments to buy individual care for their children in the community. Disabled people and their organisations in Britain took up this fight in their campaign for increased power, control and independence.

The principles of independent living maintain that disabled people have the same right to personal autonomy and choice as able-bodied people. The social model of disability underpins these principles and forms a coherent challenge to the concept of disability as an individual 'problem'. The social model of disability redefines disability as the disadvantages caused by society, which takes little or no account of people who have impairments, thus excluding them from mainstream activity.

Independent living is not necessarily about living alone or being able to do everything for yourself. It means choice over where and how to live, choice about who provides assistance and control over how, when and what they do. Independent living is about disabled people and children being able to make the same choices in everyday life as able-bodied people. It is the right to live within the community, attend local schools, have equal access to leisure and community facilities, use public transport and obtain employment, which reflects their abilities (Ratzka, 2001). Morris (1993) argues that independent living is about human and civil rights, because if disabled people do not have control over their own care needs, then they cannot hope to participate in society on an equal basis.

Following on from this there has been debate about whether the term 'independence' should be replaced with 'interdependence', on the grounds that over the course of their lives people will both give and receive care. Dependence on support therefore should be seen as an integral part of human life rather than a disaster that suddenly overtakes a person. Reconstructing dependence as a part of all people's lives at some stage removes the stigma associated with needing help. We are all interdependent upon each other.

The legislation

To facilitate the transfer of funding from local authorities to service users, the Community Care (Direct Payments) Act 1996 was implemented on 1 April 1997. This Act gave local authorities the power (but not the duty) to make cash payments to certain disabled adults, aged under 65 years, to enable them to purchase care for themselves. Prior to this it had been illegal for local authorities to make cash payments in this way, although a few got around this by making indirect or third party payments. On 1 February 2000 the legislation was amended to include older people, so that they too could receive a direct payment.

The Carers and Disabled Children Act (2000) was implemented on 1 April 2001. This extended the powers of local authorities still further to expand direct payment schemes to include people with parental responsibility for a disabled child, disabled young people aged 16/17 years, and carers of people aged 18 years and over. The legislation is permissive. It bestows a power rather than a duty on local authorities, but the Health and Social Care Act (2001) includes provision to extend the scope of direct payments still further. Subject to the implementation of the Act in 2002 the legislation will:

- require local authorities to make direct payments where an individual who requests and consents to one meets the criteria

- enable local authorities to make direct payments to disabled parents to meet their child's needs, and for rehabilitation services provided by the local authorities.

At the time of writing, a bill is in the process of going through the Scottish Parliament, which will require local authorities in Scotland to make direct payments. When these two pieces of legislation are implemented, direct payments will then become a mandatory responsibility for both English and Scottish local authorities. The government has issued both practice and policy guidance to all the direct payment legislation.

Eligibility for a direct payment

To be eligible for a direct payment an individual must meet one of the following criteria:

1. Be a disabled child or adult (see Box 1) and need

    - a community care service under the NHS and Community Care Act (1990) or
    - a service under the Children Act (1989) section 17.

2. Be a carer of a disabled adult or have parental responsibility for a disabled child (see Box 1) and provide or intend to provide substantial and regular care to a disabled individual or child who needs

    - a community care service under the NHS and Community Care Act (1990) or
    - a service under the Children Act (1989) section 17.

Box 1 Definitions of disability used for direct payment eligibility

- An adult must fit the definition used in the National Assistance Act (1948) section 29. This includes people who have physical, including sensory disabilities, learning disabilities, mental ill health, HIV/AIDS, or an illness such as arthritis.

- A child or young person must meet the definition in the Children Act (1989) section 17(11).
  This again includes physical and sensory disabilities, mental illness, learning disability or substantially and permanently handicapped by illness, injury or congenital deformity.

---

3. Be a disabled young person (see Box 1) aged 16/17 years who needs a service under the Children Act (1989) section 17.

Individuals must also

- consent to a direct payment and
- be able to manage the payment either alone or with assistance **and**
- not be subject to certain criminal justice or mental health legislation (see Box 2).

Box 2 Mental health/criminal justice exclusions from direct payments

Direct payments cannot be made to the following people:

1. Patients detained under mental health legislation on leave of absence from hospital.
2. Conditionally discharged detained patients subject to Home Office restrictions
3. Patients subject to guardianship or supervised discharge.
4. People receiving aftercare or community care as part of a care programme under a compulsory court order.
5. Offenders serving a probation or combination order subject to a requirement to undergo treatment for mental health, drug abuse or alcohol dependency.
6. People subject to equivalent Scottish mental health or criminal justice legislation.

Community Care (Direct Payments) Act 1996 Policy and Practice Guidance.

How direct payments can be used

One of the most exciting aspects of direct payments is their adaptability. Service users can use them to organise their care in a whole range of new and more effective ways. Indeed, local authorities are encouraged to explore innovative and creative options for meeting people's needs. As long as the local authority is satisfied that an individual's needs are being met, the money is being spent appropriately and, in the case of disabled children/young people, that any person providing care is a 'suitable person', then the possibilities seem almost endless.

Direct payments must be used to meet service users' assessed needs. This can be done in a variety of ways: purchasing care from an independent sector agency, respite care in a care home, meals on wheels, day care in an independent sector day centre, employing a personal assistant, etc.

They can be used to support the parents of disabled children in their caring role and to help them maintain their own health and well-being. The guidance to the legislation recognises that the responsibilities of parents caring for a disabled child are often much more arduous, because of the difficulty of accessing community based amenities. Direct payments can overcome the disabling barriers that prevent service users from accessing social and leisure facilities available to the rest of the community. They can also give parents respite. This is demonstrated in the case study in Box 3.

Box 3 Case study

Mark Denver is ten and lives with his parents and three sisters. He is a wheelchair user and requires help with all his personal care needs. Mark's father works long hours and his mother is employed part time.

Mark's parents receive a direct payment and employ a personal assistant who goes with Mark to the swimming baths with his two older sisters. The personal assistant helps Mark to get changed and to use the hoist to access the swimming pool.

The personal assistant is also employed to go with Mark to the football stadium to watch his local team.

While the personal assistant is providing support for Mark and enabling him to access community facilities, Mark's parents are able to relax and have respite from their caring responsibilities.

Direct payments enable assessed needs to be met in new ways. Parents of a disabled child could use the money to employ a personal assistant to go with their child to an after school club, to local play areas, or to provide support while they are working or looking after other children in the family. They can purchase short-term breaks for their child in a respite care home or with a suitable family, as in the case study described in Box 4.

One very important function that direct payments can fulfil for young disabled people is to assist them in the transition period from child to adult. Direct payments can be made to disabled young people

(16/17 years) in their own right to meet all or part of their assessed needs. So a young person may choose to use the local authority home care service to get him or her ready to go to school, and a direct payment to employ a personal assistant at weekends to go shopping and attend a youth club. People can have as much support as they need in order to manage their direct payment, and this gradual introduction to arranging their own affairs would assist in their development by providing a valuable learning process.

Direct payments can be used together with funding from the Independent Living Funds (ILF), provided that the service user meets the ILF criteria (see Chapter 4). This dual funding can be used to provide support for people who require large care packages, which local authorities are often unable to resource. It is an important method of enabling severely disabled people with high support needs to live interdependently within the community. See the case study in Box 5.

Box 4 Case study

Joshua Carter is eight years old and lives with his grandparents who have parental responsibility for him. Joshua is profoundly deaf and communicates by using British Sign Language (BSL). His grandparents are both hearing, although his grandmother has attended sign language classes and is now fairly proficient.

Joshua's grandparents receive a direct payment and use it to pay for Joshua to stay occasional weekends with a local deaf family who communicate using BSL. This family takes Joshua with them to the local deaf centre on Saturday afternoons to play with other deaf children and meet deaf adults.

This arrangement enables Joshua's grandparents to have a break from their caring role and for Joshua to be with people who use BSL as their first language and understand the importance of deaf culture. They can also be positive role models for him.

Box 5 Case study

Jennifer Hamilton is twenty-three and has a spinal injury following a road accident. She is paralysed from the upper chest down, with limited movement of her arms and hands. She is living with her parents at present, but has just bought a 2-bedroom bungalow where she intends to live.

Ms Hamilton's assessment shows that she needs help with all personal care tasks, including care once during the night. She needs assistance to do the shopping, cooking, cleaning, laundry and manage household finances. Ms Hamilton also needs support to enable her to access the community and socialise.

Ms Hamilton feels that a live-in personal assistant will best meet her needs. Her social worker agrees and funding is to be provided from the Independent Living Funds and a direct payment from the local authority. Ms Hamilton will use all of this funding (plus her own service user contribution) to employ two personal assistants who will live in with her on alternate weeks. (Each personal assistant will live in for a week and then have a week off.

Ms Hamilton could have chosen to employ three or four personal assistants on a rota basis, but felt the live-in option would give her more continuity of care.

Direct payments can be used to support people caring for a disabled adult. Government guidance stresses that local authorities should think creatively and focus on providing carers with what they want rather than what is already on offer. Anecdotal evidence is cited about carers being offered personal care, which they do not want, and being denied help with cleaning, which they do want. Low-level services such as cleaning, gardening and laundry are to be developed, along with the provision of mobile phones, washing machines, driving lessons, etc. It is up to individual local authorities to decide which services they are able to fund for carers. See Box 6, which details how direct payments can be used to meet carers needs.

BOX 6 CASE STUDY

Maqsood Ali Ahmad is eighty-two and has been diagnosed with Alzheimer's disease. He lives with his wife who looks after him. During the progression of the illness, Mr Ahmad lost his ability to speak English and has reverted to his first language of Urdu.

Mrs Ahmad has a direct payment and uses it to pay for a gardening company to mow the lawns and cut the hedges. She also employs a neighbour who speaks Urdu to supervise and talk with her husband on four afternoons a week. Mrs Ahmad is then able to do the shopping and have respite from the care she provides.

The legislation enables local authorities to make direct payments to individuals for the purchase of equipment, which would otherwise be provided by social services. Items such as stair lifts, bath hoists, etc. would be included in this category. Some local authorities have not yet included this part of the legislation in their direct payment schemes, perhaps because they are able to negotiate lower prices for equipment with suppliers than individuals would be able to do. However, a direct payment could be made if a more expensive item were chosen, with the service user paying the difference in price themselves.

It is important that advice is obtained to ensure that any equipment purchased is safe, appropriate and good value for money. The Disabled Living Centres sited around the country display a large range of equipment and may be able to advise.

Direct payments must not be used for permanent residential care or to purchase local authority services.

What are the benefits of direct payments?

There is now a considerable body of research that demonstrates clearly the benefits of giving disabled people money directly to arrange their own support. Direct payment users report that their care arrangements are more flexible, they offer a choice of better quality options and give them greater independence. They show much higher levels of satisfaction with their care than people using traditional services. (Glendinning *et al.*, 2000; Heptinstall, 1999; Leece, 2000)

> *'I can employ the people I like and it is satisfying to be able to pay for their services.'*
>
> *'I have the opportunity to choose when I get up, go to bed, go shopping and have recreation time, as I did before I became disabled.'*
> **Direct payment users.**

Most direct payment users choose to spend the money by employing a personal assistant, as this is the arrangement that tends to have the most advantages. One constant criticism of agency or social services support is of continually changing care staff. Service users are often visited by a series of different support workers carrying out tasks in an increasingly impersonal manner. People value reliability and consistency. They generally like to have the same known worker providing their support in the way they like it to be performed (Leece, 2001a). Recruiting your own personal assistant can fulfil all these requirements.

> *'Before I had direct payments I had about 40 home care workers in 2 years.'*

'Consistent availability of dedicated carers, the local authority workers do not stay long enough and change too often.'

'Having the same person makes a big difference. I don't have to keep explaining what I need. Having a strange person do very personal things is not pleasant.'
Direct payment users.

Individuals can recruit a personal assistant who is known to them and fits in with their routine and preferred way of being cared for. They can choose a person they trust and like.

'My personal assistants are my friends as well as my carers. One of them comes on holiday with us.'
Direct payment user.

Most direct payment schemes allow care hours to be 'banked'. So, for exmple, if a service user is assessed as needing ten hours of support each week and decides to use only eight hours in one week, the additional two hours can be added to support to be provided at a later stage. This would be useful, for example, for people needing help to learn daily living skills. A bus journey into a town to learn shopping skills may generally take too long for the support hours allocated, but by saving unused support hours it is possible for this to be undertaken. Direct payments thus provide a more flexible service, which can be tailored to meet service users' needs more precisely.

Direct payments may be used to buy care from an independent sector agency. This, of course, does not give the same level of control as recruiting your own personal assistant, but it does have an advantage over the local authority purchasing care from an agency on the service users' behalf. A direct payment user buying care from an agency and becoming dissatisfied with the services provided can simply change to another provider. This may not be so easy for a service user receiving services purchased or provided by the local authority.

Respite care may also be purchased through direct payments. This may be in the form of employing a personal assistant to stay with/care for the individual in the community while their carer has a break. Or it could be the purchase of a short stay in an independent-sector residential home. The choice of home will be up to the individual, within the limit of the direct payment made. Individuals can generally choose to make a top-up payment from their own funds if they prefer to stay in a more expensive establishment. Direct payments cannot be used to purchase respite care in a local authority home, although service users can ask for this to be provided separately from the direct payment.

The many advantages of direct payments may lead practitioners and their managers to fear that they will be far more expensive to provide, and that cash-strapped local authorities will be unable to allocate funding. The guidance to the direct payment legislation states, however, that they must be cost-effective and in line with best value. Information from research shows that payment schemes are in fact significantly cheaper than the direct service provision approach (Zarb and Nadash, 1994). Direct payments not only offer more control; they can often actually save money (Brandon and Maglajlic, 2000). They are also considerably cheaper than providing permanent residential care.

It can be seen that the benefits and possibilities for direct payments are extensive.

Are there any disadvantages to direct payments?

To examine direct payments objectively it would be wrong not to consider the disadvantages or any possible areas of concern. A study by Glendinning *et al.* (2000) has highlighted certain problems for personal assistants employed by direct payment users. The study discovered that the personal assistants were less likely to have clearly defined roles and job descriptions than staff working for agencies. They often receive low wages, have no pension provision and work in isolation without the support of other colleagues. Their working hours are frequently unspecified and they may lack training opportunities.

The study also found that some personal assistants undertake tasks that are defined as health care: physiotherapy exercise, injections, stoma and catheter care and manual bowel evacuations. Health professionals had often withdrawn because of the rationing of services or staffing problems, with these tasks being delegated to the personal assistant. In other cases personal assistants were completing the tasks at the request of their employer. While it may be convenient for service users if their personal assistants can provide care in this way, it could be argued that it is exploitation of a vulnerable group of workers. Personal assistants are often in an exposed position, they are isolated and unlikely to belong to a trade union.

Disabled people and children may also be vulnerable to abusive situations. Some practitioners have expressed concern about the possibility of unscrupulous personal assistants exploiting direct payment users. Individuals should take precautions when recruiting workers by ensuring that applicants are properly vetted (see Chapter 3).

Another area for concern is the difficulty some direct payment users have experienced when trying to recruit a personal assistant, especially in rural areas. Indeed, local authorities and independent sector agencies nationally have encountered similar problems in attracting and retaining sufficient numbers of care staff to provide the required level of services.

A recent inquiry by the King's Fund concluded that care services could be in a crisis situation within the next few years. Many private care agencies cannot compete with the flexible working patterns offered by local supermarkets.

> *'Despite advertising extensively for many months, very few people applied. Most were not suitable, for different reasons.'*
>
> *'The job centre will, of course, advertise your vacancy, as will local shops. I have only had three applications in five weeks using these methods.'*
> **Direct payment users.**

To try and improve this situation, local authorities need to ensure that direct payments are paid at a rate that enables users to compete in the job market. The rates should be high enough to enable potential employers to offer an hourly rate slightly higher than competing employers such as local domiciliary agencies, residential homes and supermarkets. Realistic recruitment costs should also be reimbursed by the direct payment.

Practitioners may be concerned about what will happen if the arrangements for support break down. For example, if a direct payment user recruits a personal assistant who then becomes ill or decides to stop working at short notice, or a service user's health may fluctuate or change suddenly. To avoid these situations turning into a crisis, detailed contingency plans to address these areas must be drawn up at the setting up stage for the direct payment. Contingency planning is discussed in Chapter 4.

So while there are a number of problem areas for direct payments, these can usually be addressed by careful planning.

Calculating the amount of a direct payment

Local authorities are at liberty to decide on the amount of a direct payment and what it is intended to cover. The guidelines do not set maximum or minimum amounts, either in the value of the payment or the support it is intended to purchase, although a local authority can set limits if it chooses to do so. A local authority is required to make a direct payment at a rate that it estimates to be the reasonable cost of an individual securing the service concerned. The amount of the direct payment therefore must be enough to cover the cost of the assessed support.

The amount of a direct payment will probably vary from one local authority to another, as will the maximum (care package limit) and minimum amounts to be spent on each person. The local authority can require direct payment users to make a financial contribution to the cost of their care package in the same way as if they were receiving traditional services. The method of calculating financial contributions made by service users are detailed in the Department of Health publication 'Fairer Charging Policies for Home Care and other Non-residential Social Services: Guidance for Councils with Social Services Responsibilities'.

Generally direct payment schemes will include the following:

1. Set-up costs – including advertising costs, stationery, insurance premiums (e.g. Employer's Liability Insurance), postage, etc.
2. Agency rate (hourly) – care purchased from the independent sector (this may be the same as the average contract price/spot contract rate charged by the independent sector).
3. Personal assistant rate (hourly) – including Employer's National Insurance contributions, holiday and sickness entitlement.
4. Retainer allowances – to cover the personal assistant's wages if the direct payment user is admitted to hospital or a care home in an emergency.
5. Respite care rate – likely to be the same as the price the local authority has agreed to pay the independent sector.
6. Day service rate.
7. Transport costs.
8. *Ad hoc* payments – training of personal assistants, protective clothing for personal assistants, further advertising costs for staff changes, associated costs, e.g. materials for training in daily living skills, etc.

The rates paid should be variable to include the higher prices charged by providers for care to service users with more complex or challenging needs.

The amount of a direct payment paid to a service user will be the amount of care hours/day services etc., detailed on the care plan multiplied by the rate allowed for that provision (see Box 7).

Box 7 Calculating a direct payment

Winifred James has been assessed as needing ten hours of personal care support each week by her social worker. She needs help to wash, dress, shop, cook a meal, etc. Mrs James has decided to have a direct payment to employ a personal assistant to provide this support. Her friend, who lives nearby, is prepared to do this work.

Her local authority direct payment rate for a personal assistant is £6.80 per hour.

Mrs James will receive a direct payment of 10 × £6.80 = £68.00 per week to employ her friend.

The direct payment rate includes National Insurance (NI) contributions, sickness and holiday entitlement, so Mrs James pays her friend £5.50 per hour, keeping the difference in her direct payment account to cover sickness pay, etc.

Direct payments must be paid into a separate bank account to ensure that they can be audited correctly (see Chapter 4). Direct payments are not classed as income and so are not liable for income tax, nor are they taken into account for social security purposes. They do not effect benefits such as Attendance Allowance, Disability Living Allowance, Income Support, etc.

The first stage in arranging a direct payment is to determine whether a service user is eligible and assess their needs.

2 The assessment process

To obtain a direct payment, a potential service user must first be assessed by social services. To meet the direct payment criteria, this assessment must identify either that an adult needs a community care service, or a child needs a service under the Children Act (1989). Carers and parents can also have a direct payment in their own right, but they must be providing a substantial amount of care on a regular basis for one of the above individuals. The assessment process, then, is of crucial importance to the process of securing a direct payment.

Many busy practitioners may fear that the assessment for a direct payment is more exacting and onerous than the assessments they complete routinely. In fact, this is not the case. An assessment, which results in the service user taking the direct payment option, is exactly the same needs-led assessment as for traditional service provision. The direct payment route can in fact involve less work for the practitioner, as he or she is not required to arrange care on behalf of the service user. Direct payment users do this for themselves (with support from a supporting organisation – see Chapter 3).

Practitioners are, however, required to assess whether service users, parents and carers are able to manage and are giving consent to receive a direct payment. They will also need to assess whether the care provided by carers and parents is substantial and regular. These issues, including a discussion of the assessment process, are considered in this chapter.

Completing a needs-led assessment

The community care reforms of the 1980s and 1990s, which culminated in 1993 in the implementation of the NHS and Community Care Act (1990), brought with them fundamental changes in the way practitioners assess and meet service users' needs. Prior to the reforms, resource or service-led assessments were completed, where needs were slotted into a 'set list' of service provision. It was common to hear practitioners talk about 'a day care assessment' or 'an assessment for respite care'. A day care assessment would inevitably result in the provision of a day centre place, almost regardless of the individual's circumstances.

The reforms brought a new system of assessment and care management which demands innovative ways of meeting service users' needs. It involves the adaptation of services to meet needs, rather than fitting people into existing service provision. A needs-led assessment identifies individual needs in partnership with the user, carer(s), advocate, etc. It is of enormous importance that this type of assessment rather than a resource-led assessment is completed for the direct payment process (see Box 8).

Box 8 Definition of assessment

'An assessment is the process of gathering and interpreting relevant information in order to understand a person and their surroundings. It is the basis for planning any action required improving or maintaining a person's circumstances. Need has been defined as 'the requirements of individuals to enable them to maintain or restore an acceptable level of social independence or quality of life...'
Care Management and Assessment: Practitioner's Guide (1991).

A needs-led assessment is vital, because it identifies service users' specific needs. This allows for care plans to be devised to meet those particular needs. A resource-led assessment, e.g. 'needs day care' can only ever provide that resource. It is easy to slip out of 'what does this person need?' into 'what have we got that he or she could have?' It is crucial that detailed needs-led assessments are completed, so that an individual's needs can be accurately translated into a direct payment. See Box 9, which demonstrates this.

Assessing service users whose needs fluctuate

Many service users will have needs that fluctuate. An example may be a person with multiple sclerosis whose ability to care for him/herself varies with the progression of the illness. A needs-led assessment should be completed which estimates the number of care hours required over perhaps a 6–8 week period. The individual then uses the number of hours they need each week. Remaining hours are 'banked' and used as required (see Box 10). Should the needs of the service user increase significantly, making the estimated figure too low, a reassessment must be completed.

Box 9 A needs led assessment

John Davis has learning disabilities and lives at home with his father. John is able to care for himself in terms of washing/dressing/using the toilet, etc., but lacks the knowledge and confidence to complete household tasks, as his father has always taken care of them.

John wishes to move into a home of his own, but is worried that he will not be able look after himself. An advocate has been working with John to help him identify what he wants to do. A social worker is also involved and she has completed a needs-led community care assessment to determine John's needs.

The assessment identified that John needs help to learn daily living skills such as preparing food, cooking, making a shopping list, shopping, cleaning, laundry, managing a household budget, using a bank account and paying bills.

John's needs could be met by a day service place, where training in daily living skills is provided (likely cost to the local authority would be £27 per day).

However, John would prefer to attend his local college, which runs a similar course on two mornings a week. He has decided to have a direct payment to purchase a support worker from an agency to facilitate his going out into the community, paying bills, using a bank account and doing shopping. The support worker will also assist him to put his college training into practice, by helping him to do some cleaning, cooking and laundry at home.

John will be supported to manage the direct payment by the supporting organisation, (see Chapter 3).

John will need 3 hours of support per week.

His local authority direct payment rate for agency care is £8 per hour.

John's direct payment will be £24 per week (less any service user contribution).

Box 10 Assessing fluctuating care needs

Jake Davenport is sixteen years old and has a condition that fluctuates. Sometimes he is able to wash and dress himself ready to go to school, but on other days he is too weak and needs assistance. He has a direct payment and chooses to buy support from a private agency.

Mr Davenport's assessment looked at a typical 8-week period of his life. Over that 8-week span the assessment identified that he needed on average, 3 hours of support each week.

Sometimes only 1–2 hours are used each week, with the remaining time being 'banked' in Mr Davenport's direct payment account. At other times, when he is feeling less strong, he uses 4 or 5 hours per week. This averages out to the assessed figure of 3 hours per week.

Assessing disabled children and young people

The direct payment guidance advises that a practitioner from children's services should always be involved in any assessment of disabled children and young people. The assessment should follow the procedure in 'The Framework for Assessing Children in Need and their Families'. This provides a format for assessing a child's needs and the abilities of it's parents to respond to these needs, within the context of the family and the community. The assessment should be multidisciplinary involving the child, it's parents, and health and educational professionals. An independent advocate may also be involved.

Disabled young people aged 16/17 years can have a direct payment in their own right, provided that they consent to the payment and are able (with support) to manage it. There may be situations where a practitioner considers a young person is 'able to manage and consents to' a direct payment, yet the parents disagree, for whatever reason. In circumstances such as this, where conflict is involved, the role of the independent advocate to promote the young person's views is likely to prove invaluable.

The guidance to the Carers and Disabled Children Act is clear in its response to such areas of disagreement. If the young person wishes to have a direct payment and the local authority considers they are 'consenting and able to manage' then the views of the young person should have precedence over their parent's views. The overriding requirement is whether the provision of the direct payment will promote and safeguard the young person's welfare.

Assessing carers

Carers have had the right to an assessment of their needs ever since the implementation of the Carers (Recognition and Services) Act (1995). The Carers and Disabled Children Act (2000) extends and increases these rights. To be eligible for an assessment under the new Act, carers must be providing or intending to provide a substantial amount of care on a regular basis for a disabled adult. The Act gives carers the right to an assessment even where the person they care for has refused an assessment or has refused the delivery of services. The Act gives local authorities the power to offer carers services (or direct payments) to:

- support their caring role
- to help carers maintain their own health and well being.

It is important that practitioners advise all carers who are identified during an assessment for a cared for person, that they have the right to request a carer's assessment. Many carers will not be aware that this right exists.

A carer's assessment will often take place at the same time as the assessment for the cared-for person, although it can take place at a different time. All parties should be given the facility of separate assessments if this is preferred. The same practitioner will generally undertake both assessments, although, in situations where there is conflict, it may be appropriate for another worker to be involved. A friend or relative of the carer can be present during the assessment and an independent advocacy service should be offered.

The guidance to the Act stresses that carers' assessments should focus on outcomes, e.g. what it is that the carer wants to happen. It provides a series of modules to lead the practitioner through the assessment to find out about the caring relationship from the carer's perspective. Similar questions are reproduced in Box 11.

Some potential service users may refuse an assessment, which can cause difficulties. The legislation states that, to obtain a direct payment, the carer must be providing care to individuals assessed as needing a community care service. Where people do refuse to have an assessment, it will often still be clear that they would be eligible for a service. There will be occasions, however, where it is more difficult to judge whether the individual would be eligible or not. In these circumstances, the guidance suggests that corroboration can be sought from other professionals involved, such as the carers' GP. In the absence of suitable verification, the local authority may still decide to complete a carer's assessment and provide services/direct payment to the carer in any case.

Box 11 Carers' assessments

Does the carer feel that he or she has a choice about caring?
Is the carer willing and able to continue providing care?
How much time is spent caring?
Can the carer get a break?
Is the carer well?
Does the carer undertake any tasks that put him/her at risk?
Is the carer stressed?
What would happen if the carer were suddenly taken ill?
Does the caring role have an impact on other relationships?
Are there any accommodation difficulties?
Are finances a problem?
Does the carer want to stay in or return to work?
What support does the carer get at present?
How does the carer see the future?
What does the carer want to happen?

A Practitioner's Guide to Carers' Assessments under the Carers and Disabled Children Act 2000.

The carer may request that the cared-for person is not told about their request for a carers' assessment. Good practice demands that practitioners are truthful about the source of referrals. Should the carer be determined on this, then unless there is a risk of real harm to them or the person they care for, the guidance states they will not be eligible for an assessment or services/direct payments under the Act.

It is important that individuals, who are often under a great deal of pressure from their caring responsibilities, should have full information and enough time to think through the implications of receiving a direct payment. The time for this should be built into the assessment process.

Assessing young carers

The Carers and Disabled Children Act guidance is clear on its stance regarding young carers. It states that they should not be providing a substantial amount of care on a regular basis. Support should be provided by social services for their disabled parent(s), to avoid this happening. For practitioners, this causes a dilemma. Clearly, the reality is that many children are providing large amounts of care for their parents. Indeed, the National Carers Strategy (1999) identifies young carers as potentially the most disadvantaged of all children, and estimates that there are between 20,000 and 50,000 in Britain. Many of these receive no support at all from either statutory or voluntary agencies.

To avoid young carers 'slipping through the net' and not being provided with adequate support, there should be effective liaison between practitioners from adult and children's services. The difficulty for local authorities is that many are obliged to impose maximum limits to care packages for adults, because of funding shortages. A disabled parent who has reached the maximum limit of their care package may be compelled to spend their own money to purchase the extra support required, or rely on care provided by their child. An application to the Independent Living Funds (see Chapter 4) may help to resolve these situations.

With regard to direct payments, the guidance stresses that there will be few situations where making a direct payment will be the most appropriate way of meeting the needs of young carers. The responsibilities involved in arranging care may well be too much for a young person already undertaking caring responsibilities. On the few occasions where a direct payment is provided to a young carer, local authorities must be satisfied that this will be the best possible outcome for the young person.

Direct payments may be useful where a disabled parent has rejected contact with social services and refuses services. Providing a young carer with the money to purchase his or her own support may be more acceptable to the parent, as it requires less contact with statutory agencies.

Children's services should always be involved in any assessment of a young carer. They are eligible to receive services under section 17 of the Children Act (1989) and should be assessed using the guidance in 'The Framework for Assessing Children in Need and their Families', (especially paragraphs 3.61–3.63).

Assessing people with parental responsibility

During any assessment of a child with disabilities, parents should be advised by practitioners that they have the right to request an assessment of their ability to provide and continue to provide care for their child. To be eligible for an assessment under the Carers and Disabled Children Act (2000), parents must be providing or intending to provide a substantial amount of care on a regular basis. Given the enormous amount of work that most disabled children generate, it seems very likely that the majority of parents will meet this criteria.

Direct payments can be made to parents to:

- meet the assessed needs of their disabled child
- to support parents in their caring role
- to help parents maintain their own health and well-being.

Before a direct payment can be made, the local authority must be satisfied that the arrangements in place will safeguard and promote the welfare of the child.

Defining 'substantial and regular'

To obtain an assessment under the Carers and Disabled Children Act, parents and carers must be providing or intending to provide a substantial amount of care on a regular basis. There is, however, no definition of these terms in the guidance, and it is up to individual local authorities to decide their meaning.

Some local authorities may choose to define them in terms of an average weekly figure, such as 20 hours per week. There are dangers in this, though, as there are bound to be situations where the needs of the carer or parent justify an assessment, even though they are carrying out care duties for less than the stipulated weekly amount. The guidance considers that it is not only the time spent each week in caring, but also the *impact* that the caring role has on carers. Various factors should be taken into account. Is the carer/parent getting enough sleep? Are they concerned that they might have to give up work? Is their health being affected by their caring role? Are other relationships affected? Can the carer/parent get out and about? Do they have time for themselves? Can they care adequately for other children?

There are a number of situations where carers and parents providing care for only short periods of time should be eligible. They may have ill health or be very old. They may be providing care from a distance and spending many hours in travelling time. The emotional and mental impact of providing support should not be ignored; caring for a person with dementia or a child with challenging behaviour for even a few hours can be exhausting.

In defining substantial and regular, practitioners should ensure that they consider:

- Is the caring role sustainable?
- How large is the risk of the caring role becoming unsustainable?

There are many complex situations that will require unravelling. Care may be provided by more than one carer, with each providing a substantial amount of care on a regular basis. All are eligible for an assessment. Carers may live across council boundaries. The guidance states that in those circumstances it is generally the cared-for person's home authority that is responsible for the carer's assessment and service provision. People with disabilities may live together and provide some care for each other. The guidance refers to people in this situation as 'interdependent'. Practitioners will need to complete a thorough needs-led assessment that details accurately the care each person is giving and receiving.

Consent to a direct payment?

Assessing whether an individual is able to give consent to a direct payment may be problematic at times, especially for practitioners working with service users who have a learning disability or dementia. A direct payment can only be made with the consent of the person concerned, so it is important that this is resolved satisfactorily. It is made more difficult because of the lack of legal clarity about the ability to consent, which is rarely ever tested in a court of law.

The issue of consent causes enormous concern and is probably the main factor for the reluctance of many local authorities to fully embrace direct payments for people with learning disabilities. There has been a very low take-up of direct payments nationally for people with learning disabilities (see Chapter 4). The ability to consent, however, was never intended to be a barrier hindering people in their desire for greater independence and choice. Making the decision to have a direct payment should be seen as a process, and not a test that an individual has to pass. Indeed, the White Paper 'Valuing People: A New Strategy for Learning Disability for the 21st Century' stresses the government's commitment to developing ways of enabling greater numbers of people with learning disabilities, including the most severely disabled, to make choices and express their views. The White Paper reiterates that 'direct payments are highly effective in enabling people with learning disabilities to gain greater control over their lives, because they can choose how they want their support needs met'.

Practitioners therefore need to develop ways of enabling people with learning disabilities to make choices and demonstrate their consent. The White Paper talks about the increased use of advocacy, including self-advocacy and the person-centred approach to enable people with learning disabilities to make known their wishes and aspirations. A person-centred approach reflects the needs and preferences of individuals. It means putting people at the centre of the planning for their lives by:

- listening and learning about what people want from their lives
- helping individuals to think about what they want now and in the future
- family, friends, practitioners and service providers working together with the person to make this happen.

Person-centred approaches are ways of making sure that services are more responsive to users' wishes. It is an approach that can enable people with high support needs, who may not be able to speak up for what they want, to make their views known. The White Paper introduced 'Disability Partnership Boards' to develop plans for person-centred planning. The plans are to be called 'A Framework for Person Centred Planning'.

Values into Action considers the 'supported decision making model', can also aid individuals to make decisions and give or withhold consent, (Edge, 2001).

This model makes the following assumptions:

- all human beings communicate
- all human beings express choices and preferences about their lives
- these choices and preferences are the building blocks of decisions
- when people's choices and preferences lead to action, this shows that individuals are controlling their own lives, even if they need substantial help to make their choices happen.

The model indicates certain crucial factors that aid the process of decision-making for people with learning disabilities:

- provide accessible information (for example, the Department of Health produces 'An easy guide to direct payments for people with learning disabilities')
- give people enough time to decide
- reduce the formalities
- respect the way people communicate and use imaginative ways to ensure effective communication (pictures, photographs, simple and appropriate language, multi-media, etc.)
- enable people to make decisions in their own environment
- reduce the pressure; make things more relaxed
- don't take initial uncertainty as an automatic refusal. It should instead prompt an examination of the areas of concern, so that solutions can be offered
- involve the individual's supporters (friends, peers, family, advocates, etc.)
- have collective responsibility for recording the evidence of choices.

Assessing whether people are able to consent to a direct payment when they have a deteriorating cognitive disability such as dementia is also a challenge. Methods from the supported decision-making model could prove helpful in enabling choices to be made. People with dementia can be provided with a direct payment via an enduring power of attorney, although the individual must have consented to the direct payment at the time they had the capacity to do so, as an attorney cannot give consent on another person's behalf. Bearing this in mind, it will be useful for practitioners to find out the wishes of people who are in the early stages of dementia, by providing them with information about direct payments. Individuals can then give consent while they are still able to do so.

Either the local authority or an individual can decide at any time that they no longer wish to continue with direct payments. It is then the responsibility of the local authority to arrange or provide services.

Able to manage

Local authorities should only make direct payments to people they consider able to manage them (alone or with assistance). They can refuse to make a direct payment to anyone they determine unable to manage it. The guidance is quite clear that local authorities must consider each person individually and not make blanket decisions about whole groups of people. For instance, local authorities cannot offer direct payments to older people, but exclude everyone diagnosed with dementia. Each person must be assessed individually.

It is important to remember that people receiving direct payments do not have to manage them alone or in isolation. They can have as much or as little help as is required. There are many examples of individuals who need almost total assistance with their direct payment, but still manage to control it. The crucial element is not whether someone can complete income tax forms, write cheques and manage their workers, as support for this can be provided. It is whether the individual receiving the payment is controlling the situation and making decisions about how the money is spent.

Assessing an individual's ability to manage the direct payment may be difficult in certain situations. The guidance stresses that the decision about a person's ability to manage should reflect the complexity of the task required. For example, managing a large care package is likely to require more skill than a package of a few hours only.

Direct payments can be paid for part or all of the assessed needs. People can opt to have a mixture of provision depending on their preferences and how their needs are best met. This could be helpful in enabling people to gain the skills to manage a direct payment gradually. It may also be useful for young people in the transition period from childhood to adult responsibilities.

It is important not to view the need for support to manage the direct payment as a problem. People should be offered as much or as little support as is required. This can be given by the agencies that support direct payment schemes. Many support agencies, for example, offer a 'salary service' where they complete the paperwork involved, calculate tax and National Insurance payments, complete Inland Revenue returns and so on, on behalf of the direct-payment user. Ongoing support should be discussed and organised as part of the setting-up process of the direct payment.

The decision about an individual's ability to manage should not be made in isolation from the support networks available. Family, friends, neighbours or advocates can all provide the necessary support to enable an individual to manage a direct payment. The costs involved can be detailed in the care package and paid for in the payment. For people whose ability to manage is in doubt, a time-limited trial period could be provided with a lot of support, or a direct payment being made for a small part of the care package only, to enable the individual to be as independent as possible.

Supporting service users to enable them to access direct payments is an important part of the process. It is discussed in much greater detail in Chapter 3.

3 Supporting people to use direct payments

Support services for direct payments

Providing support for service users and carers to enable them to access direct payment schemes is crucial. Indeed, the Department of Health (DOH) considers that the development of a support service is essential to the success of a direct payment scheme. It is important to remember that individuals can have as much or as little help as they require. To provide this help, the guidance to the legislation suggests that local authorities form partnerships with local voluntary organisations. Some local authorities fund local groups of disabled people to provide support. There are many Centres for Independent Living throughout Britain which provide information and have a supporting function for direct payments. A list of these can be obtained from the National Centre for Independent Living (see page 63).

Supporting organisations can provide a whole range of assistance. For example, information about direct payments, advice regarding employment legislation, help to draft contracts of employment, job specifications and job adverts, help to short-list and interview applicants, provide rooms for interviews, offer peer support, training for personal assistants, help with form filling, a salary service and so on. The support offered can be the deciding factor in empowering individuals to take the direct payment option. Many people are worried about the responsibilities involved in becoming an employer. They are concerned that social services will abandon them and they will be left to manage alone. Supporting organisations should be involved from the outset to provide information and reassure people that support will be readily available.

Support to manage a direct payment can also be given by a professional employment adviser or an accountant, a person's family, neighbours, colleagues and friends. It can be written into the care plan (bearing in mind the restrictions on employing close family) and paid for by the direct payment.

Purchasing care from an agency

Probably the simplest way for service users to spend their direct payment to arrange their care is to purchase it from an independent sector agency. There are a number of advantages to using an agency and it may provide the answer for people who want the independence of a direct payment, without the responsibility of becoming an employer. It could also be helpful in situations where an individual's ability to manage a direct payment is in question, or where they lack the initial confidence to manage an employee. Using agency care may give people the self-assurance to become employers themselves at a later date.

> *'I am not prepared to be considered an employer by the government. I do not have the time and wish only to deal with agencies and self employed people.'*
> **Direct payment user.**

The agency providing care is the employer of the worker and manages all the responsibilities of tax, National Insurance contributions, training, recruitment, etc. Cover for sickness and holidays of the usual care worker will be provided by the agency. Domiciliary care agencies are required by the Care Standards Act (2000) to register with the National Care Standards Commission who have a regulatory function.

There are, of course, disadvantages too. Using agency care may not give individuals as much control over the way their support is delivered as employing a personal assistant directly for themselves would do. The service provided will be to the standards set by the agency, which may well be lower than the standards a person would set for their own care. Using an agency is likely to give the direct-payment user less freedom.

Individuals employing their own personal assistants can also use agency care in their contingency plans to provide care when their personal assistant is unavailable due to sickness/holidays, etc.

Recruiting a suitable personal assistant

Recruiting a personal assistant is the most popular use of direct payments and it has many advantages in terms of control, flexibility and independence for the employer. When making a direct payment to an adult, a local authority must be satisfied that the payment will be used to meet the person's needs. The money can be used to employ anyone who is eligible to work, other than those people specifically excluded by the legislation (see next section). However, with children and young people the situation is more complex. Local authorities must not only be sure that assessed needs are being met; they must also be satisfied that the personal assistant employed to do so is a 'suitable' person. The local authority can refuse to make a direct payment if it is to be used to employ a person who is unsuitable.

The Police Act provides the base for criminal records checks and provision is made by the Care Standards Act (2000) to allow parents and young people to ask a local authority to carry out criminal records checks of potential employees. These can be undertaken using the Protection of Children Act (1999) via the Criminal Records Bureau (CRB), which came into operation in March 2002. The CRB is the government's new 'one stop shop' for checking criminal records. There have been some difficulties with the CRB, however, and local authorities should use existing arrangements for these checks if there are still operational problems.

A criminal record check which reveals no convictions still does not guarantee that a person is suitable to provide care for a child or young person. The guidance recommends that parents are vigilant and take the following precautions:

- ask for two references and check them with the referee
- if there are any doubts do not employ the person
- clarify where the child may be taken and who will be present
- ask about and check out other members of the personal assistant's family, if the child is to have contact with them
- does the personal assistant smoke and is this a problem, e.g. would the child be subjected to passive smoking?
- take notice of what the child communicates about the care they receive
- watch for unusual or regressive behaviour, especially in children who are non-verbal.

Vulnerable adults should also take appropriate precautions when recruiting support staff. Research by Barnes (1997) found that many older people were concerned for their safety and worried about the risk of employing people who had not been 'vetted' by the local authority. Local authorities can carry out criminal record checks for adult direct-payment users on potential personal assistants. Interviewees can also be asked to provide certificates which they can obtain from the police, detailing any previous convictions (the cost is about £10 for a basic check, at the time of writing).

> *'Although you can get an idea of what people are like at an interview, I wouldn't, of course know if they had a criminal record. I have to give people a key to my home. I think they should be vetted.'*
> **Direct payment user.**

Recruitment of personal assistants has been a problem for direct-payment users nationally, especially in rural areas. Bearing this in mind, local authorities should set direct-payment wage rates for personal assistants that are competitive in the local job market. For example, wages need to be slightly higher than those offered by competing employers such as domiciliary care agencies, residential homes and local supermarkets, to enable direct-payment users to recruit suitable, quality staff. Wages must also comply with the Minimum Wage Legislation, which, at the time of writing, is set at £3.50 per hour (18–21 years) and £4.10 (22+ years). In certain situations, to aid recruitment, local authorities will need to give serious consideration to direct payment users being able to employ close family.

Employing family

The Community Care (Direct Payments) Act, section 1(4) prevents people from using their direct payments to employ their partner or a close relative living in the same house. In addition, they cannot use their direct payment to employ a close relative living elsewhere; or another person living in the same household as the direct payment user. However, a local authority may decide to make an exception to this rule, if it is satisfied that this is the most appropriate way of arranging the relevant service. See Box 12 for the definition of close relatives.

Box 12 Definition of close relatives

A close relative is defined as: a parent, parent in law, aunt, uncle, grandparent, son, daughter, son-in-law, daughter-in-law, stepson or daughter, brother, sister, or the spouse of any of these,

A partner is the other member of a married or unmarried couple.

Interestingly, grandchildren and cousins are not included in the list, and so may be employed by direct-payment users, as long as they are not living in the same household.

Community Care (Direct Payments) Act 1996 Policy and Practice Guidance

---

This regulation is not intended to prevent individuals employing a live-in personal assistant; the restriction operates where the relationship is mainly personal rather than contractual. For example, when the individuals concerned would be living together despite any employment connection.

For practitioners, the importance of the restriction is the effect it may have on direct-payment users. The general thinking is that, if relatives are employed, direct-payment users may find it more difficult to achieve genuine independence. But for some people this takes away choice about how they use their direct payment. One relative of a direct-payment user who wished to employ her said: 'We were told we couldn't do this. We feel this is very unfair, because it is dictating who she can and can't employ, and also expecting me to provide care for free.'

The restriction can disadvantage people from ethnic minority communities. In Muslim communities, women prefer to be cared for by other female family members, and this may cause people to refuse help from social services. Research indicates that direct payments are failing to attract people from ethnic backgrounds and the limitation on employing family members may account for some of this, (Butt *et al.*, 2000). Local authorities can agree that non-resident family members can be employed if it is the most appropriate way of securing the relevant services. In Coventry, for example, direct-payment users can employ close relatives if there are cultural or religious reasons.

There are other situations where practitioners should consider this. Older people with dementia may be more likely to accept help from known and trusted relatives than from new support staff, of whom they have no long-term memory. Deaf people and parents of deaf children may wish to employ a personal assistant whose first language is sign language and who is knowledgeable about deaf culture. Recruiting a deaf person as a personal assistant may be difficult, and family members could be considered. Recruitment problems generally could be an area where employment of family should be considered. Some local authorities agree that close relatives can be employed in rural areas, where recruitment can be particularly hard.

Recruitment and employment information

Organisations supporting direct payment schemes have expertise in the recruiting and employing of personal assistants and will be able to help individuals who wish to spend their direct payment in this way. It is likely, therefore, that most social work practitioners will not need to provide this level of support to their service users. The following sections regarding recruitment and employment issues are included to increase practitioners' knowledge in case they need this information, and for practitioners who work in areas where support is not provided by specialist organisations.

Creating a job description/person specification

It is important to decide the specific tasks the personal assistant will be required to perform, and what their duties/responsibilities will be. The starting point will be the service users' needs-led assessment and care plan, which will detail all the requirements. The views of the service user about the type of care they want should be paramount. The job description should list exactly what is required from the personal assistant: what their responsibilities will be, the hours involved, whether they are required to live in, to work on a rota system or be a single worker, the salary paid, etc. This will help potential applicants to decide whether they are able to do the job and if they wish to apply. A good job description should include:

- the main purpose of the job
- the main tasks involved – stated specifically rather than in vague terms. For example, 'cooking and meal preparation' rather than 'dealing with domestic matters'.

Having completed a job description detailing the requirements, it will then be possible to profile the person required to fill the job; this is the person specification. Person specifications should consider:

- the length and type of experience required
- education, training and qualifications needed
- skills related to the job
- personal qualities and attitude required.

Contract of employment

A contract of employment is an agreement entered into by an employer and an employee. It defines the terms and conditions of the employment and details the responsibilities and duties of the employer (see Box 13). As soon as an employee starts work, a contract exists between both parties, even if there is nothing set down in writing. It is a legal requirement that, within two months of starting work, an employee is given a written statement setting out the principal terms and conditions of the job. Both the employer and the employee should sign the contract.

The contract of employment is a legally binding document. It is unlawful for either party to alter the terms and conditions unless there is mutual agreement. Should an employer wish to change the terms of the contract – for example, a change in the work undertaken – they should discuss this with the employee. If the employee objects to the change, the employer could decide to terminate the contract by dismissing the worker. The statutory notice or wages in lieu of notice would have to be given. The employer could then recruit another worker or employ the dismissed worker with new terms and conditions. A dismissed employee could take the case to an Industrial Tribunal if he/she felt there had been unfair treatment, and there was a record of at least two years' continuous service.

Advertising

Once the tasks, duties and conditions of service have been decided, the potential employer can start to advertise for the personal assistant.

Box 13 Contract of employment

Contracts should contain the following:

- name of employer and employee
- date of appointment
- basic rate of pay (together with rates for bank holidays, unsociable hours and weekends)
- rates for travel expenses
- method of paying wages and travel expenses (e.g. cash, cheque, into a bank account)
- holiday entitlement
- procedure for taking holidays
- place of work
- hours of work
- job description
- notice period required
- length of probationary period (if any)
- employer's responsibilities (e.g. wages, National Insurance contributions)
- sick pay arrangements
- disciplinary and grievance procedure (as a 'small' employer it is not necessary to include these, but it is good practice to do so)
- types of behaviour classed as gross misconduct (e.g. theft, fraud)
- variations that may be needed (e.g. requiring an employee to undertake different types of work at times).

Most direct payment schemes include funding for advertisements, although this will probably only extend to local rather than national press. Advertisements in local newspapers are usually the most effective method of recruitment, but can be expensive, especially if repeat adverts are required.

Local job centres will display adverts on their boards free of charge, as will some supermarkets and shops. Local college notice boards and certain newsletters may also be effective. It will be more useful to advertise in publications read by specific groups of people if a specialist personal assistant is required. For example 'British Deaf News' if the personal assistant needed is a deaf person who uses sign language. There are newspapers published for ethnic communities too. Adverts can be placed on the Internet, and 'word of mouth' could be effective, as many people recruit friends and neighbours. The advert should briefly detail the following items:

- nature of the job
- pay
- qualifications required
- geographical area involved
- hours
- employer's phone number and a box number to contact
- request for applicants' CV
- date of interview.

Interviewing

Interviewing can be quite stressful, and it will probably be helpful for the service user to have a supporter present. This could be a friend, relative, social work practitioner, another direct payment user, etc. The interview could be held in the individual's home or other suitable premises, such as a room in the local social service office, library, community centre, etc.

Interview questions should be prepared beforehand. Depending on the employer's requirements these could include:

- Why do you want the job?
- What have you got to offer?
- What previous experience do you have?
- What relevant qualifications do you have?
- Do you have a current driving licence?
- Do you have a car?
- Do you have any health problems?
- Are you a smoker?
- What are your interests and hobbies?

All candidates should be asked the same questions, to give them an equal opportunity to present themselves, and to enable comparisons to be made. Notes can be taken of the responses made, or a scoring system can be used on each question. Candidates should provide references and it is advisable to check these either in writing or by telephone. Employers should avoid unfair discrimination, but they can choose someone who meets their needs or their way of life. For example, a gay man may want a gay personal assistant to help him to access certain venues; a female with personal care needs may prefer these to be undertaken by another woman; a deaf child may need a personal assistant fluent in British Sign Language, and so on. Information can be obtained from Equality Direct, an organisation set up by the Advisory, Concilliation and Arbitration Service (ACAS) to give free confidential advice on any equality issue in the workplace. Telephone/textphone 0845 600 34444, or www.equalitydirect.org.uk.

Peer support by other direct payment users who have already recruited staff could prove invaluable. They could provide information and advice based on their own experiences. Training in interviewing skills can also be given. This could be funded as part of the setting-up process of the direct payment.

When the direct-payment user has decided which candidate he or she wishes to employ, it is probably best to offer the job subject to a probationary period, of perhaps three months. This will give the employer time to decide if the personal assistant is really suitable. The length of the probationary time should be stated in the contract of employment.

PAYE and National Insurance contributions

The management of an employee's PAYE and National Insurance (NI) contributions can be quite daunting. It is for this reason that many organisations supporting direct payment schemes operate a payroll or salary service. These ensure that the relevant paperwork is completed, the employee's salary is correctly paid, and their contributions are deducted accurately. Some direct payment schemes may not have a supporting organisation and it is worth contacting the nearest Centre for Independent Living to investigate whether they can offer a payroll service. Some Councils for Voluntary Services may be able to help, or this service could be purchased from an accountant or bookkeeper, with the cost built into the direct payment.

Some direct-payment users may prefer to be responsible for managing this part of the direct payment themselves, and during the tax year they will need to:

- deduct the correct amount of PAYE from the employees' pay
- calculate the correct amount of NI contributions they and their employees need to pay
- keep a record of the employees' pay, PAYE due and NI contributions due
- make monthly or quarterly payments of the total NI contributions and PAYE due.

Employers should register with the Inland Revenue as a new employer (New Employers' Helpline 0845 607 0143 or 0845 602 1380 (textphone). The relevant information and forms will then be issued. There is also an Employers' Helpline (0845 714 3143), which gives information about PAYE and NI contributions, including Maternity Pay and Statutory Sick Pay. Employees earning less than £89 per week from (April 2002) are not required to make NI contributions or PAYE. The employer should still register as a new employer, however, and must keep a record of the employee's earnings. New employees should give their employer their P45 when they start work. If they do not have a P45, employers should issue them with a P46 (available from the New Employers' Helpline).

Personal assistants who are self-employed are responsible for their own PAYE and NI contributions. However, employers should seek clarification about an individual's employment status from their local Inland Revenue office (see leaflet IR56, 'Employed or Self-Employed', for information). The leaflet can be obtained from the Employers' Helpline. Personal assistants can get a letter from the Inland Revenue to prove that they are registered as self-employed. This is important because, if a personal assistant does not make the required contributions, the 'employer' may be held liable.

Employers can operate payroll systems on their own computers, and there are special computer programmes available to do this. Anyone purchasing a payroll programme should check that it has the Inland Revenue's Payroll Standard Kitemark.

Direct-payment users who purchase care from an independent sector agency are not responsible for the collection of tax and NI contributions of the agency workers; agency care staff are employees of the agency.

Statutory Sick Pay

Direct payment users who are employers will need to be aware of the rules regarding Statutory Sick Pay (SSP), in case their employees are unable to work because of illness. To qualify for SSP an employee must:

- be aged 16 or over, and under 65 years
- have average weekly earnings of not less than the Lower Earnings Limit (currently £75 per week) prior to becoming ill. They do not need to have paid any NI contributions
- have been incapable of working because of illness for a least four consecutive days (including weekends and public holidays).

An employee can self-certificate for the first seven days of their illness, but after that they should provide an employer with a doctor's note. The Inland Revenue has produced a form (SC2), which employees can use to self-certificate themselves. This is available from the Employers' Orderline on 0845 764 6646.

SSP is paid in the same way as wages are usually paid, and is liable for tax and NI contributions. It is paid at a daily rate depending on the number of qualifying days in a week. Qualifying days are the days of the week the employee usually works. SSP is not paid for the first three qualifying days in a period of sickness (waiting days). The daily rate of SSP is the weekly rate of £63.25 divided by the number of qualifying days in the week, beginning with Sunday. SSP can be paid for a maximum of twenty-eight weeks in a single period or linked periods of sickness.

Employers should issue employees who are not eligible for statutory sick pay with form SSP1 after the fourth day of illness.

Detailed information about SSP is in the SSP manual for employers (CA30) and SSP tables (CA35) from the Employers' Orderline.

Maternity rights and Statutory Maternity Pay

All pregnant employees, regardless of length of service, whether working full or part time, are entitled to paid time off for antenatal care. The rate of pay is the rate the employee is normally paid. They are also entitled to eighteen weeks' ordinary maternity leave. During ordinary maternity leave the employee must continue to receive all contractual benefits (e.g. holiday entitlement, use of mobile phone, etc.) except wages or salary.

Employees who have completed a year's continuous service with their employer by the eleventh week before the expected week of confinement are eligible also to receive additional maternity leave. This runs from the end of ordinary maternity leave up to the end of the twenty-ninth week after the baby is born. Contractual benefits continue during additional maternity leave too.

Employees must not return to work for at least two weeks after childbirth, and this can be longer depending on the type of employment. This is known as compulsory maternity leave.

The employee must produce a certificate from a registered doctor, midwife or health visitor confirming the pregnancy. Employers can ask to see an appointment card documenting that antenatal appointments have been made.

Employers must pay Statutory Maternity Pay (SMP) to employees who are eligible to receive it. To be eligible for SMP, an employee must:

- have been in continuous employment for at least 26 weeks by the end of the 15th week before the baby is due
- still be pregnant at the 11th week before the baby is due, or have had the baby
- have average weekly earnings of not less than the Lower Earnings Limit (at the time of writing, £75 per week). They do not need to have paid any NI contributions
- have produced medical evidence of the date the baby is due (form MATB1)
- have stopped work. SMP cannot be paid for any week in which an employee has worked.

SMP is paid for a maximum of 18 weeks. For the first six weeks it is paid at 90 per cent of the employee's average wage. For the remaining 12 weeks it is £75 per week (from April 2002).

All employers can recover 92 per cent of the SMP paid to an employee, and small employers (such as direct-payment users) may be able to recover 100 per cent of the SMP paid plus 5 per cent compensation. Detailed information about this and SMP generally is available in the SMP manual for employers (CA29) and SMP tables (CA36) available from the Employers' Orderline.

The employer should give form SMP1 to employees who are not eligible for SMP. This will enable them to claim Maternity Allowance from the Benefits Agency.

SSP and maternity pay would be managed by the payroll or salary services for individuals choosing to access this.

Holiday entitlement

The Working Time Regulations implemented in October 1998 gives employees entitlement to a minimum of 4 weeks' paid leave per year. A week's leave is calculated on the time that an employee usually works, so if an employee works five days a week they will be entitled to a minimum of 20 days leave per annum, while a part-time employee working 10 hours a week is entitled to 10 hours' leave in lieu of every one week's holiday, giving a total of 40 hours each year.

Personal assistants must be employed continuously for 13 calendar weeks to qualify for the full leave entitlement. Should an employee cease work before completing a full year, then their leave entitlement is proportional to the amount of time they have worked. So an employee working for only 6 months before leaving will be entitled to 2 weeks' leave in that leave year. Further information about this can be obtained from ACAS on 0121 456 5856.

Employers may decide whether to pay employees for public and bank holidays.

From January 2002 parental leave has been extended to parents of children who were under five years of age as at 15 December 1999. For more information see the Department of Trade and Industry website at www.dti.gov.uk/er/parental-leave.htm.

An employee's leave entitlement and the procedure for their taking holidays should be detailed on the contract of employment. See Box 13 on page 37.

Health and safety legislation

There are a number of legislative requirements employers must usually take into account, and these are detailed in the following regulations:

- Health and Safety at Work Act (1974)
- Management of Health and Safety at Work Regulations (1992)
- Manual Handling Operations Regulations (1992).

This legislation deals with the assessment of health and safety risks to employees and how to avoid these risks to protect them. The legislation, however, does not apply to individuals directly employing their own personal assistants to work in their home, although it is good practice for employers to provide employees with a safe working environment. Where direct-payment users purchase care from an agency, then the agency, as the employer, is responsible for the health and safety of the worker.

There may be a dilemma with regard to achieving safe working practices for employees and the rights of disabled people to be cared for in the way they prefer. The National Centre for Independent Living (NCIL) have highlighted this issue for people who wish to be lifted manually rather than by a hoist (NCIL, 2001). Some local authorities are interpreting the Health and Safety legislation to mean 'no lifting' and then placing this requirement on direct-payment employers, even though, as previously stated, the legislation does not in fact apply to them. The Disability Rights Commission argues that 'no lifting' policies are likely to be unlawful. They may also be a breach of disabled people's rights under the Human Rights Act (1998) article 3 (not to be subjected to inhuman or degrading treatment).

The NCIL considers that it is unrealistic to try to achieve an entirely risk-free zone for disabled adults and children (or indeed anyone). There should be a careful analysis and balancing of risks, which take into account both the rights of disabled people and the need to create a safe working environment. Appropriate training and support should be provided to enable employees to operate safely while upholding the independence of direct-payment users.

For further information contact the Health and Safety Executive Infoline 08701 545500, or www.hse.gov.uk

Insurance

Employers have a responsibility to insure employees against accidents or injury occurring during their employment. This may be a personal assistant falling down the stairs, burning themselves while cooking dinner, food poisoning from eating food provided by their employer, tripping over while carrying the shopping, etc. Employers need to take out insurance to provide for these situations.

- Employers Liability Insurance covers accidents or illness involving employees. This is sometimes provided in household contents policies, but this generally does not cover accidents away from the home. It may therefore be necessary to use a company specialising in this type of insurance. (Fish Insurance is the leading specialist, on Freephone number 0500 432141.) Local authorities must include the cost of this insurance in the direct payment

- Public Liability Insurance covers injury or harm to the public by the personal assistant during their employment
- house buildings (if owner-occupied) and contents insurance, as the personal assistant may cause damage to property
- car insurance if the personal assistant is to drive the direct-payment user's car, or increasing the personal assistant's insurance to cover business use, if they are to use their own car.

Stakeholder pensions

Individuals who employ five or more personal assistants, where at least one is earning more than the Lower Earnings Limit for NI contributions, must designate a stakeholder pension provider unless:

- they already offer an occupational pension scheme to all employees
- they offer a contribution of at least 3 per cent of earnings into the employee's personal pension plan.

Employers must give their workers details of the provider, and the employees then decide whether they wish to save for a pension in this

---

Box 14 Gross misconduct

Gross misconduct is not defined in law, but ACAS consider it to take the form of acts that involve a serious breach of contract. It is behaviour resulting in loss of trust and confidence. Employers should decide the type of behaviour that will constitute gross misconduct and this should be detailed in the contract of employment. Examples of gross misconduct could be:

- theft
- fraud
- breach of confidentiality
- verbal abuse
- physical abuse
- being at work under the influence of alcohol or drugs (other than those obtained under prescription).

Employees dismissed because of gross misconduct should be paid any holiday pay due.

National Centre for Independent Living (www.ncil.org.uk/sacking).

---

way. Deductions for stakeholder pensions will need to be made via the employees' salaries. Building societies, banks and insurance companies all offer stakeholder pensions. For a full list of providers, see www.stakeholder.opra.gov.uk.

Dismissing a personal assistant

There may be times when direct-payment users are not satisfied with the care their personal assistants are providing and wish to dismiss them. Employing people on a probationary or trial period initially may help to avoid this happening, but unsuitability may not become apparent within this period. Great care should be taken in these situations, as employees who are unfairly dismissed can claim compensation; it is advisable therefore to seek specialist legal advice. Direct payment support organisations should also be able to help. An employer can dismiss an employee if all the following conditions have been met:

- the employee is given the correct amount of notice (unless there is gross misconduct – see Box 14)
- the employer has acted reasonably in deciding to dismiss the employee
- the reason for the dismissal is fair (see Box 15).

The correct amount of notice to be given is one week for people employed for at least a month. Employees who have worked for more than two years should receive two weeks' notice plus an additional week for each extra year worked, up to a maximum of twelve weeks.

Box 15 Dismissal that is fair

A dismissal is generally fair if:

- the employee's job no longer exists (redundancy)
- the employee is not capable of doing the job
- the employee's conduct is unacceptable (e.g. failing to come to work repeatedly without good reason)
- a legal requirement prevents the employee from doing their job
- another substantial reason.

National Centre for Independent Living (www.ncil.org.uk/sacking).

---

4 Making direct payments work

Direct payments enable disabled people to have more power, choice and autonomy over their lives. They are flexible and provide the means to create innovative solutions for meeting people's care needs. Research shows they are cheaper than traditional service provision (Zarb and Nadash 1994, Brandon and Maglajlic 2000)) and direct payment users consistently report far higher levels of satisfaction about the way they receive their social care.

Yet despite all this, statistics collected by the Social Service Inspectorate (SSI) in September 2000 show that in England only 3,742 people were receiving a direct payment. By Autumn 2001, whilst this had increased by almost 45%, still only 5,423 people were accessing direct payments, even though the legislation was changed in April of that year, to enable the inclusion of parents, carers and young disabled people. The latest figures from the SSI 2002 show that the total number of people receiving direct payments has risen to just 7,882. The take up rate also varies widely depending on an individual's disability (see box 16).

Almost every local authority in England now has a direct payment scheme in place, although some have not extended their schemes to all

---

BOX 16 STATISTICS FOR PEOPLE RECEIVING A DIRECT PAYMENT IN ENGLAND

Direct payment totals September 2002

Physical disabilities	5459
Sensory disabilities	159
Learning disabilities	736
Mental health	132
Older people	1032
Carers	95
Young carers	3
Disabled children	38
Carers of disabled children	228
Total	**7882**

Social Services Inspectorate.

---

groups of disabled people, children or carers. Figures for Scotland indicate that they are further behind in terms of implementing direct payments. A study by the Scottish Executive (Ridley and Jones, 2002) found that only 16 out of the 32 local authorities were operating a direct payment scheme, although others were operating 'third party schemes'. Only 213 people in Scotland are accessing direct payments, only 70 more people than two years ago. Almost all the recipients have a physical disability, with just two having mental ill health.

So why is it that so few people are accessing direct payments?

Changing the culture

Research by the National Centre for Independent Living found that one of the most important factors for making a direct payments scheme a success is the willingness of practitioners to offer the option to individuals. Care managers who are 'enthused' by direct payments and see them as an exciting, viable and innovative way forward are more likely to suggest them as a positive choice to service users.

Yet many practitioners will be feeling unsure and resistant to the idea of giving individuals cash to arrange their own care. Glasby and Littlechild (2002) express concern about the ability of social service departments to achieve the significant changes required by the direct payment legislation. They argue that, in recent years, social work has involved arranging services for vulnerable people, and giving people the cash overturns more than 50 years of social work practice. Social workers are just not used to dealing with money.

Practitioners may be concerned about vulnerable people being exploited and what will happen if things go wrong. The shift in control from the local authority to service users may result in practitioners feeling unsure of themselves and insecure. Because of this, practitioners may not be offering direct payments to certain groups of service users they feel would be at risk, such as people with a learning disability, mental ill health or dementia. They could have mistaken beliefs that older people don't want to be bothered and are happy to have care organised for them, even though research indicates that older people value their autonomy just as much as younger people and are very keen to maintain their independence.

Direct payments do require a change of culture for both local authorities and practitioners. There needs to be a shift in the way risk and control are approached, with an acceptance that service users have the right to take risks to achieve a greater degree of responsibility and control in their lives. The identification of any hazards together with systems to combat them (such as contingency plans, monitoring, legal agreements, independent advocacy, involving wider networks and so on) should help to reassure practitioners and assist in the change of ethos required.

To improve the numbers of people being offered and taking up the option of direct payments it is crucial this organisational and cultural change takes place.

Contingency planning

Planning for emergencies and unforeseen events is vital for the smooth running of individual direct payments. However good the care arrangements are there will be times when they break down or go wrong. This will be especially important for people with fluctuating conditions such as multiple sclerosis or mental health needs.

Having an effective contingency plan in place is also likely to reassure practitioners and make their life less stressful. Local authorities do have a responsibility to provide services if they are not satisfied that an individual's needs are being met. So if adequate care is not being provided in an emergency situation, the local authority still has overall responsibility to provide or organise care services.

Contingency plans should be discussed and agreed at the time the direct payment is arranged. Plans should cover alternative arrangements for direct-payment users' care if their personal assistant becomes ill, leaves the job with little notice, books a holiday at short notice, etc. They should also detail care provision should the needs of the employer change. Sickness and holiday pay for the usual personal assistant should be included within the direct payment hourly rate paid for personal assistants (see Chapter 1). Types of alternative provision could include:

- recruiting a personal assistant who is able to offer flexible working hours, so they can provide extra support if needs fluctuate
- care could be provided by a named friend, neighbour or family member (taking into account the restrictions on employing family – in emergency situations the local authority may wish to agree that employing a family member is the most appropriate way of meeting the service user's needs)
- recruiting two personal assistants who are flexible and can cover for each other
- using an independent care agency. This could be agreed in advance with the agency
- using local authority home care workers – the direct payment cannot be used to pay for these, but care can be provided as direct service provision
- some agencies supporting direct payment schemes can arrange emergency back-up support or shared personal assistant schemes
- respite stay in an independent sector care home. This may be difficult to arrange at short notice, and would involve the direct-

payment user phoning care homes to check vacancies. Respite care can be provided in local authority homes as direct service provision

- co-operative schemes agreed by groups of direct payment users where personal assistants can be shared in times of emergency.

Contingency planning will not avoid emergencies developing, but they will stop them turning into crises.

Box 17 Contingency planning

Winston Jackson has learning disabilities and uses his direct payment to employ a personal assistant for 12 hours a week. The personal assistant enables Mr Jackson to access his local community by assisting him to use the local swimming baths, shops, cinema and cafés. In an emergency, Mr. Jackson's cousin, who works part time, has agreed to work for him and provide the required care.

Bernard Cheung has mental health needs. He has a direct payment that he uses to employ a personal assistant to encourage him to do his shopping and cook a main meal. The personal assistant is employed for 10 hours a week. In an emergency, Mr Cheung has decided he would prefer the local authority to provide his care with their own home care service. It has been agreed that his personal assistant will telephone the social services duty officer if an emergency occurs.

Monitoring and reviewing direct payments

When an individual chooses to receive a direct payment, the local authority's responsibility to arrange a service is removed, as long as it is satisfied that the person's needs are being met. If the local authority is not satisfied, then its responsibilities towards the service user remain the same as if a direct payment had not been made. To ensure that direct payment users' care arrangements are meeting their needs, methods of monitoring/reviewing should be put in place that are consistent with the arrangements for direct service provision.

A monitoring/reviewing schedule could be:

- a meeting to check that arrangements are satisfactory 6–8 weeks after the direct payment has started
- a review after 6 months

- annual or 6-monthly reviews depending on the nature of the situation.

Some direct-payment users may wish to have as little communication with the local authority as possible, seeing this contact as diminishing their independence. Arrangements should be sensitive to this while still ensuring that checks are in place. People who have been managing their care arrangements successfully for some time or who have stable conditions may only require annual reviews. New direct-payment users with fluctuating illnesses or need very large packages of care are likely to need more frequent monitoring.

People whose ability to manage a direct payment is in doubt could be encouraged initially to have a 'mixed package', with part of the care being provided by a direct payment and part by direct service provision. This would enable closer monitoring to be undertaken by local authority workers to determine that the service users' needs are being met. This process should be fully explained to the service users, so that they are aware that care workers have a monitoring role.

Local authorities should also set up financial monitoring procedures to enable direct payments to be audited. The Chartered Institute of Public Finance and Accountancy have issued guidance on this (www.cipfa.org.uk). Users of direct payments will need to keep financial records of their care transactions, and help with this can be provided by organisations supporting direct payment schemes.

Involving people from minority ethnic communities

There is a great deal of research indicating that people from minority ethnic communities are not accessing either mainstream social service provision or direct payments (Butt *et al.*, 2000; Evans and Banton, 2001). This research has identified some of the barriers for people from minority ethnic communities, which act to prevent them from becoming involved with social services. The impact of structural, cultural and individual oppression are clearly shown:

- existing services/direct payment schemes are often inappropriate; e.g. they do not meet language or cultural needs
- practitioners may use stereotypes to avoid providing services, e.g. considering that people from ethnic communities receive all the help they need from their families
- little awareness of cultural issues within organisations
- many funding organisations do not recognise the need for specific work with disabled people from minority communities
- restrictions on funding may mean that the focus is either on race or disability rather than on both together

- the stigma attached to disability within some black communities, which may be caused by the dearth of disability awareness-raising undertaken in these communities compared to that among the white population
- lack of accessible information, outreach and advice targeted specifically at minority ethnic communities.

The flexibility of direct payments offers great potential for the inclusion of marginalised groups of people in society. People from minority communities can use direct payments to employ personal assistants who understand their cultural needs and background. Instead of attending non-specialist day centres where there may be language barriers to full inclusion, a personal assistant from the user's community can enable disabled people from minority communities to access their local community groups, shops and religious festivals.

There are a number of strategies practitioners can use to aid the inclusion of people from minority ethnic communities into direct payments schemes. See Box 18.

Box 18 Some strategies for including people from minority communities in direct payment schemes

- involve disabled people from minority ethnic communities in the consultation process and setting up of direct payment schemes
- provide accessible information in a variety of formats and appropriate languages, ensuring concepts are translated meaningfully. Community groups could be used as access points for information
- provide advocacy and outreach (with workers from the relevant minority community if possible)
- encourage peer support
- recruit bilingual workers to direct payment schemes and supporting organisations
- ensure workers have an understanding of the impact of racism and oppression by providing training
- work with other organisations which have expertise on race and disability
- develop good links with community leaders.

Involving people with mental health needs

People with mental ill health have been able to use direct payments since the legislation was first implemented in 1997. The figures from the SSI, however, indicate that only 132 people with mental illness in England have taken up the option and this probably represents the lowest take-up rate for all the groups of eligible service users. The figures for carers and disabled children are lower in number, but they have been eligible for a direct payment only since April 2001.

There are some exclusions from direct payment eligibility for individuals with mental illness, such as people subject to guardianship or detained under mental health legislation (see Chapter 1).

Some people with mental ill health will have fluctuating care needs, and the flexible nature of direct payments enables these needs to be met very effectively. (See the case study in Box 19.) For people with mental health needs who require encouragement to care for themselves, adequate monitoring arrangements should be put in place to ensure that their needs continue to be met. The case study in Box 19 also demonstrates how a personal assistant can undertake this monitoring role by visiting each morning to check whether support is required. Service users may be able to undertake this role themselves, or family, friends, neighbours, etc could do so.

Box 19 Case study

Anurada Devi suffers from mental ill health. She has had post-natal depression since the birth of her baby five months ago. On good days, Mrs Devi is able to care for herself and her baby, but at other times she needs encouragement and help to shop, prepare food for herself and the baby, and do the laundry.

Mrs Devi's needs-led assessment has estimated that she needs on average 9 hours of care each week. She has opted to receive a direct payment to employ her friend, who speaks Hindi. Mrs. Devi's English is good, but she prefers to speak Hindi, which is her first language. Mrs Devi's friend is also of the same religion (Hindu) and understands which foods can and cannot be eaten by people of their religion. She calls in to see Mrs Devi every morning to find out if she is needed. This 'pop in' visit has been included in the estimated care hours.

The fluctuating nature of Mrs Devi's illness means that some weeks she uses more than the allocated 9 hours of care, and other weeks she uses less. On the occasions when she uses less, the remaining hours are 'banked' to be used as necessary at a later date.

To be eligible to receive a direct payment individuals must be able to manage the payment. Each individual can have as much or as little assistance as necessary to do this (e.g. to organise recruitment and pay staff, etc.), but that person must be the one who is making the choices and is controlling how the money is spent. People with mental ill health may vary in their ability to appear in control, especially if at times they are distressed. To help with this problem, a service user could write advance directives for workers to follow when their employer appears not to be in control. An advance directive would detail, for example, what a personal assistant should do if the direct payment user appears withdrawn, depressed or unwell. It would state emergency contact numbers and what to do if the situation turns into a crisis.

There are other methods of enabling people to control their direct payment and these are explained in the next section.

User-Controlled Independent Living Trusts, Enduring Power of Attorney, Service Brokerage and Court of Protection

A direct payment may be made via a third party acting as an agent who will receive and manage the payment, while acting on the wishes of the direct payment user. It can also be made by a User-Controlled Independent Living Trust. A Trust may be beneficial where there is nobody suitable to take on the role of agent, or if there is a need to involve more people. A Trust would usually be made up of 3–4 trustees, who could be family, friends, solicitor, accountant, etc. The trustees should understand and carry out the wishes of the direct payment user.

People can be provided with a direct payment via an Enduring Power of Attorney, although the individual must have consented to the direct payment at the time they had the capacity to do so, as an attorney cannot give consent for a direct payment on another person's behalf. An Enduring Power of Attorney is a legal document by which someone appoints one or more persons to act for him or her should they become incapable of acting for themselves in the future.

It is necessary to use a solicitor to set up both a Trust and an Enduring Power of Attorney.

The Court of Protection can be used to administer the financial affairs of a person who is unable to manage for themselves. The Court will appoint a Receiver, who can be a relative, friend, solicitor, accountant, etc. If there is no appropriate person to be Receiver, then the Court will appoint a Public Trustee from the Public Trust Office. The Receiver or Public Trustee can then administer the direct payment. The Public Trust Office can advise on this process.

There may be a misconception that individuals who have their affairs managed by the Court of Protection do not have the capacity to consent to a direct payment. This is, in fact, incorrect, as people cannot be deemed incompetent to make a decision about one area in their life simply because they are considered incompetent in other areas (Ryan and Holman, 1998). Each decision about capacity can only relate to a particular decision-making aspect, so that an individual may have their financial affairs under the jurisdiction of the Court of Protection, but still be able to make choices and decisions about how their care is provided and so control a direct payment.

Independent Service Brokerage schemes exist in some areas of the country. Their role is to determine how individuals want their care to be provided, and to facilitate it. Brokers can act to find the most appropriate provision and stimulate the development of the required service. They can also act as advocates for people.

Involving people with learning disabilities

The take-up rate for direct payments has been disappointingly low for people with learning disabilities. From an estimated 1.2 million people in England with learning disabilities, only 736 currently receive a direct payment. Much of the reluctance of local authorities and practitioners to include these service users probably stems from their concerns around the 'consent and manage' eligibility conditions.

Yet the spirit of the direct payment legislation is to be as inclusive as possible, and it is very important that too-rigid interpretations of the ability to consent and manage, which exclude many people with learning disabilities, are avoided, as the legislation is clearly intended to include them. Practitioners need to use methods of enabling service users to demonstrate their consent (see Chapter 2) and ensure the provision of as much support as is required to manage the direct payment. Many people with learning disabilities have shown that, with the right support, they can exercise control over direct payments and make choices about how their care is delivered.

Again, methods such as User-Controlled Trusts, the Court of Protection, etc. can be used to enable people to manage their direct payments.

Practitioners may need to explore the provision of independent advocacy, self-advocacy schemes and awareness/training in direct payments for people with learning disabilities, to improve the accessibility of their direct payment schemes. Values into Action (telephone 020 7729 5436) may be able to assist with this.

People with HIV or AIDS related illness

The SSI statistics for direct payments does not contain a category for people with HIV or an AIDS-related illness, so it is impossible at the time of writing to determine how many are accessing direct payment schemes.

The National Centre for Independent Living (NCIL) together with the National AIDS Trust have been involved in a project to look into HIV and direct payments. They have found that, because direct payments are a relatively new way of organising care, few people with HIV have, as yet, used them, although a number are receiving money from the ILF to purchase care.

Direct payments have just as much to offer people with HIV as other service users. They provide a flexible arrangement for people whose illness fluctuates, and the control of being able to employ a personal assistant to suit an individual's lifestyle. User-Controlled Trusts and Enduring Power of Attorney can facilitate the continued use of direct payments should the direct payment user's health deteriorate.

The NCIL cites situations where people with HIV are in hospital because they cannot care for themselves at home. They could use a direct payment to fund their own personal assistant, which would enable them to return home. In these situations practitioners will need to liaise closely with both the health authority and the ILF to obtain the maximum funding.

Direct payments and the Independent Living (1993) Fund

It is important that practitioners are aware and make full use of the Independent Living Funds (ILF), as they can be a valuable way of getting more funding for people to live autonomously in the community. Direct payments can be paid at the same time as funding from the ILF, and people may be eligible for an award from the ILF if they:

- receive at least £200-worth of services (or direct payment) per week from the local authority, net of any charges made to the service user
- are aged at least 16, and under 66 at application
- receive the high rate care component of the Disability Living Allowance
- need more care at home than they can afford and the local authority can provide in order to live in the community rather than in residential care
- be able to live at home for at least 6 months
- receive income support or income at the same level or less than income support
- live alone or with people who are unable fully to meet their care needs
- have savings/capital jointly with their partner of less than £18,500 (from 8 April 2002).

Direct payment users who meet all the above criteria are eligible to make a claim from the ILF and a successful award can substantially increase the amount of funding individuals have to pay for care. The maximum the ILF can currently award is £375 a week. The award is made to the individual, who can then use the money to employ a personal assistant or use agency care, etc. in the same way as with direct payments.

Health funding for direct payments.

Many individuals will have health as well as social care needs, and direct payments have the potential to provide people with truly 'joined up' care. The Health Act (1999), section 67, allows funding provided by a health authority towards a package of care through a section 28A transfer to be used to make a direct payment. This would enable individuals to purchase integrated care.

Research shows that some personal assistants are undertaking tasks defined as health care, such as: injections, stoma and catheter care, physiotherapy exercises and so on. Yet there is little evidence that health authorities are contributing towards direct payments. This means that social services effectively are subsidising some health care provision. Practitioners should engage in open discussion with health authorities to ensure that health funding is provided for people with nursing needs.

Access to work scheme

Many disabled people are in paid employment, including being self-employed. They can obtain their costs for personal assistance associated with their work from the Access to Work Scheme. This scheme can be accessed via the Department of Employment Disability Service Teams. It covers such things as: a note-taker or reader for a person who has a visual impairment, an interpreter or lip speaker for a deaf or hard of hearing person, a support worker if practical help is required either at work or getting to and from work, and specialist equipment.

Direct payments can be used in conjunction with the Access to Work Scheme, and practitioners, together with service users, will need to liaise with Department of Employment staff to agree the most effective package.

5 Conclusion

The benefits of direct payments for disabled adults and children, older people, young people, parents and carers have been demonstrated clearly. They give people control over their own lives and extend the opportunity to do the things able-bodied people take for granted. Being able to pay for their own support releases people from the treadmill of someone else deciding when and how their care should be provided. Direct payments offer people independence and choice.

There are enormous advantages for practitioners too. They now have the facility, probably for the first time ever, to meet service users' needs effectively. Instead of providing services that the local authority deem to be appropriate and have on offer, social workers can empower individuals and facilitate truly personalised care packages that actually work. Practitioners are at last in the position of being able to provide what service users really want.

Direct payments are not for everyone, and there are disadvantages. Most difficulties can be overcome, though, with careful thought and planning. There has to be a change of culture in social services with practitioners accepting a less controlling role and embracing disabled people's rights to take risks in their life.

It is hoped that this book will achieve its objectives of giving practitioners the knowledge and information to feel confident about offering direct payments and helping service users to access them successfully, and it will have enthused practitioners with a burning desire to enable people to be independent and take control of their own care. Because social workers are the key to direct payments, they are the gatekeepers, and without them disabled children and adults probably won't get the chance to be independent and make choices in their lives.

'I have been released from my prison by my direct payment. I am back in charge. I am happy and I am free.'

Bibliography and further reading

A Practitioner's Guide to Carers' Assessments under the Carers and Disabled Children Act (2000).

Brandon, D. and Maglajlic, R. (2000) 'Direct payments: the information deficit', *Working with Older People*, pp 26–7.

Butt, J., Bignall, T. and Stone, E. (2000) *Directing Support; report from a workshop on direct payments and black and minority ethnic people*, Joseph Rowntree Foundation, York.

Department of Health Social Services Inspectorate, (1991) *Care Management and Assessment: Practitioner's Guide*, HMSO, London.

(2000) *Carers and Disabled Children Act, Policy and Practice Guidance.*

(1999) *Caring about Carers: a national strategy for carers*, HMSO, London.

1996 *Community Care (Direct Payments) Act, Policy and Practice Guidance.*

Department of Health (2002) *Planning with People: Towards Person Centred Approaches*, Department of Health, London.

Department of Health *An Easy Guide to Direct Payments*, Department of Health, London.

Department of Health *A Guide to Receiving Direct Payments*, Department of Health, London.

Edge, J. (2001) *Who's in Control? Decision-making by people with learning difficulties who have high support needs*, Values into Action, London.

Fruin, D. (2000) *New Directions for Independent Living: Inspection of independent living arrangements for younger disabled people*, Social Services Inspectorate.

Glasby, J. and Littlechild, R. (2002) 'Independence pays? Barriers to the progress of direct payments', *Practice: The Journal of the British Association of Social Workers*, 14(1).

Glendinning, C., Halliwell, S., Jacobs, S., Rummery, K. and Tyrer, J. (2000) *Buying Independence: Using direct payments to integrate health and social services*, Policy Press.

Hasler, F., Campbell, J. and Zarb, G. (1999) *Direct Routes to Independence: A guide to local authority implementation and management of direct payments*, Policy Studies Institute.

Heptinstall, D. (1999) 'Direct payments offer older people hope of greater empowerment', *Working with older people*, 3(1), pp 23–5.

Leece, J. (2000) 'It's a matter of choice: making direct payments work in Staffordshire', *Practice: the Journal of the British Association of Social Workers,* 12(4), pp 37–47.

Leece, J. (2001a) 'Directing support: direct payments and older people', *Generations Review: The Journal of the British Society of Gerontology,* 11(3).

Leece, J. (2001b) 'Changing Direction: Direct payments and disabled children', *Representing Children: A Quarterly Journal for all those concerned with the Rights and Welfare of Children and Young People,* 14(4), pp 215–25.

Morris, J. (1993) *Independent Lives: Community care and disabled people,* Macmillan, London.

NCIL (National Centre for Independent Living) (2001) *Background Paper on Health and Safety, Risk Management and Independent Living for Disabled People,* www.ncil.org.uk/health_safety.asp.

Ratzka, A. (2001) *What is Independent Living?,* National Centre for Independent Living (www.ncil.org.uk).

Ridley, J. and Jones, L. (2002) *Direct What: A study of direct payments to mental health service users,* Scottish Executive Central Research Unit (www.scotland.gov.uk).

Ryan, T. and Holman, A (1998) *Able and Willing? Supporting people with learning disabilities to use direct payments,* Values into Action, London.

Zarb, G. and Nadash, P. (1994) *Direct Payments for Personal Assistance,* Joseph Rowntree Foundation, York.

Useful contacts

Advisory, Conciliation and Arbitration Service (ACAS) 0121 456 5856, www.acas.org.uk

Chartered Institute of Public Finance and Accountancy website www.cipfa.org.uk

Disability Discrimination Helpline 08457 622633

Department of Trade and Industry www.dti.gov.uk/er/maternity.htm and www.dti.gov.uk/er/parental-leave.htm

Equality Direct (ACAS) telephone and textphone 0845 600 34444, www.equalitydirect.org.uk

Health and Safety Executive Infoline 08701 545 500, www.hse.gov.uk

Inland Revenue New Employers' Helpline 0845 6070143

Inland Revenue Employers' Helpline 0845 7143143, (textphone) 0845 6021380

Inland Revenue Employers' Orderline 0845 7646646, fax 0870 2406406

Inland Revenue website www.inlandrevenue.gov.uk – click on to 'Employers'

National Centre for Independent Living, 250 Kennington Lane, London SE11 5RD, telephone 020 758 1663, minicom 020 7587 1177

National AIDS Trust, New City Cloisters, 188–196 Old Street, London EC1V 9FR

People First, 299 Kentish Town Road, London WC1X 9DB, telephone 020 7485 6660

Values into Action, Oxford House, Derbyshire Street, London E2 6HG telephone 020 7729 5436, www.demon.co.uk/via/